Dukaı

GW00983798

The Dukan Diet Attack Phase

Recipe Book 7 Day Meal Plan

For The First Phase Of The

Dukan Diet

Written By

Sharon Stone

Sharon Stone

This document is geared towards providing exact and reliable information in regards to the topic and issue covered. The publication is sold with the idea that the publisher is not required to render accounting, officially permitted, or otherwise, qualified services. If advice is necessary, legal or professional, a practiced individual in the profession should be ordered.

- From a Declaration of Principles which was accepted and approved equally by a Committee of the American Bar Association and a Committee of Publishers and Associations.

The information provided herein is stated to be truthful and consistent, in that any liability, in terms of inattention or otherwise, by any usage or abuse of any policies, processes, or directions contained within is the solitary and utter responsibility of the recipient reader. Under no circumstances will any legal responsibility or blame be held against the publisher for any reparation, damages, or monetary loss due to the information herein, either directly or indirectly.

Respective authors own all copyrights not held by the publisher.

The information herein is offered for informational purposes solely, and is universal as so. The presentation of the information is without contract or any type of guarantee assurance.

The trademarks that are used are without any consent, and the publication of the trademark is without permission or backing by the trademark owner. All trademarks and brands within this book are for clarifying purposes only and are the owned by the owners themselves, not affiliated with this document.

Table of Contents

Introduction

I want to thank you and congratulate you for buying the book, "The Dukan Diet Attack Phase Recipe Book.

This book contains proven meal plans and recipes for the first, protein only, stage of the Dukan Diet, designed to help you lose weight and to maintain a healthy weight for life. The book forms part of a series of five books – the first covers all stages of the diet in detail – while the remaining four cover the stages with suggested meals and recipes to help you along the way.

Thanks again for buying this book, I hope you enjoy it!

Chapter 1

The Dukan Diet Attack Phase Planner and Recipes

Welcome to the Dukan Diet Plan Attack Phase Meal Planner and Recipe Book. This book is part of a series which provides an overview of the Dukan Diet and how to implement it effectively along with recipe books for the stages of the diet. The first book covers each stage of the diet and should provide you with a framework to structure your diet and put it into action. The remaining books in this series look at each phase and tackle the biggest problem that many people face with the Dukan Diet – i.e. what on earth to cook!

Processed foods – and too much food – combined with sedentary lifestyles are largely to blame for the rapidly expanding waistlines of many of us in the Western World. Cooking your own food, from scratch, is the best way to ensure you live and eat healthily. Not everyone has as much experience as they might in this area and because the Dukan Diet is most effective if you prepare your own meals this can be a problem. In each of the books in this part of the series we aim to provide you with simple recipes, that are easy and fun to prepare and shouldn't challenge even those who have previously been a stranger to the kitchen!

The Attack Phase is the shortest, but most challenging, of the four phases of the Dukan Diet. In this phase all but protein is eliminated from your diet. It can last between five and seven days – longer for some individuals but normally seven is a good guideline. Cooking meals that contain no vegetables and no starchy foods is quite a challenge for most of us. However, the phase is short enough and if you prepare in advance you will get through this phase successfully. Because the focus is on Pure Protein (PP) in this phase it offers the least variety in terms of ingredients. However, with a little clever cookery and the help of this book, you should find that your Attack Phase need not be boring. The Dukan Plan does allow you to eat as much as you like of the allowed foods – and be aware that in order to combat snacking and cravings – eating regularly and ensuring that you get three meals a day is essential.

We hope that this book will help you to find inspiration and also assist you in getting through the first phase of the Dukan Diet.

Chapter 2

Breakfast Meal Plans and Recipes

Breakfast is an important meal – it fires you up for the day and provides you with the energy you need to get moving and stay active. During the Dukan Diet, especially in the attack phase, the lack of carbohydrate can mean that you will feel low on energy. Oat bran is included in every stage of the diet and the morning is a good time to include this slow release energy food into your meal.

Suggested Meal Plan

Day One

1 Boiled Egg

1 piece Dukan Toast (1/2 tbsp oat bran) made with just egg whites

Low fat Yogurt

Day Two

Vanilla Oat Bran Porridge (1 ½ tbsp oat bran) no eggs

Day Three

Scrambled Eggs with Bacon in Dukan Style Sandwiches

Day Four

1 Chocolate Oat Bran Muffin(1 tbsp oat bran) 1/3 egg

Yogurt

Day Five

Chocolate Oat Bran Cereal (1 ½ tbsp oat bran) ¼ egg

Day Six

Fromage Frais with reduced fat, no sugar added, cocoa powder and sweetener (non-fructose)

Day Seven

2 small Dukan Cinnamon Oat Bran Pancakes (1 ½ tbsp oat bran) made with just egg whites

Yogurt

Breakfast Recipes
Oat Bran Toast

Ingredients (Makes 4 Pieces)

- 3 tablespoons of oat bran

- 2 tablespoons of low fat yogurt

- 1 egg or 2 egg whites

Method

1. Beat the egg whites in a bowl to add air.

2. Stirring well, add the yogurt and oat bran.

3. Heat a non-stick pan and add a dash/squirt of oil and then place four round egg rings in the pan.

4. Divide the mixture between the rings and level off each one.

5. When first side is cooked, remove from the rings and cook the other side.

6. Flatten the pieces of toast by applying light pressure for a few seconds

7. Grill on both sides until brown and enjoy hot or cold.

Vanilla Oat Bran Porridge

Ingredients (makes 2 servings)

- 3 tablespoons of oat bran

- 125 ml of low fat milk.

- Vanilla essence to taste

- Sweetener (non-fructose) to taste

Method

1. Place the oat bran and milk in a small microwaveable bowl and heat on high for 45 seconds.

2. Remove from the microwave and add the vanilla essence and sweetener (non-fructose) to taste.

3. Allow to stand for a few minutes for the oat bran to soak up the milk

4. Return to the microwave and cook on high for a further 45 seconds.

Chocolate Oat Bran Cereal

Ingredients (makes 4 servings)

- 6 tablespoons of oat bran

- 3 teaspoons of of low fat, no sugar added, cocoa powder

- 1 whole egg and 1 egg yolk

- Sweetener (non-fructose) to taste

Method

1. Place oat bran and cocoa in a bowl mixing throughly together.

2. Beat the eggs in another bowl along with the sweetener and then add to this mixture to the oat bran mixture.

3. Create small balls with this mixture and then lay on baking paper on a baking sheet.

4. Press down lightly on the top of each ball with a fork.

5. Place in a preheated oven at 375 degrees F for approximately 15 minutes.

6. Place on a wire tray to cool.

7. The cereal can be served with low fat milk or with low fat yogurt.

Sharon Stone

Oat Bran Pancake

Ingredients

- 1 beaten egg (or 2 beaten egg whites)

- 1 1/2 tablespoons of oat bran

- 1 1/2 tablespoons of zero fat quark or fromage frais

- Low fat (skimmed) milk if needed

- Seasoning or sweetener of choice

Method

1. Mix together the egg, oat bran and quark or fromage frais with the seasoning (or sweetener) of your choice, adding a little milk to thin the mixture if required.

2. Add a few drops of oil to a non-stick frying pan and wipe with a paper kitchen towel.

3. Add the mixture to the pan and cook on a medium heat until bubbles have formed on top of the pancake.

4. Turn the pancake and continue to cook until nicely browned.

These pancakes can be made in larger batches and can be frozen or kept in the refrigerator for up to a week.

Sharon Stone

Chocolate or Cinnamon Oat Bran Muffins

Ingredients

- 6 tablespoons of oat bran
- 4 teaspoons of reduced fat, no sugar added cocoa powder
- 2 eggs
- 6 tablespoons of zero fat yogurt
- 1 teaspoon of baking powder
- Sweetener to taste

Method

1. Mix all the dry ingredients in a bowl.
2. Add the yogurt and eggs and whisk until smooth.
3. Add sweetener to taste.
4. Divide the mixture equally between 6 paper muffin cases in a muffin tray.
5. Bake in a preheated oven at 350 degrees F for 15 to 18 minutes.

Cinnamon Oat Bran Muffins

Use the recipe above but

1. Omit the cocoa powder and instead add 1 1/2 teaspoons of cinnamon.

2. Reduce the quantity of yogurt to 5 tablespoons.

Scrambled Eggs and Bacon in Dukan Style Sandwiches

Ingredients (Serves 2)

- 2 Oat Bran Galettes (see recipe below)

- 1 pack of turkey bacon rashers

- 4 eggs

- 4 tablespoons of skimmed milk

- Dill or tarragon (or your preferred herbs)

- Salt and Pepper

Method

1. Prepare two pancakes using the oat bran galette basic recipe, set aside on a plate and cover with foil to keep them warm

2. Now prepare the scrambled eggs mix: break 4 eggs into a bowl, add the skimmed milk and gently break the eggs with a fork, stirring lightly. Season with salt and pepper and add a pinch of dried dill, tarragon or your preferred herb.

3. Spray a non-stick pan with vegetable oil and heat. Add the egg mixture, let it set slightly and use a

spatula to scrape the eggs from the sides of the pan and fold them over into the middle of the pan. Continue folding the mixture over until the eggs are cooked but still moist

4. Spray a second non stick pan with vegetable oil spray, heat it up and gently fry the turkey rashers

5. Once the turkey is cooked, place the rashers over the pancakes, top up with the scrambled eggs and fold the oat bran galettes to form two sandwiches.

Basic Oat Bran Galettes

Ingredients (Serves 2)

- 2 eggs (whole or whites only)

- 3 tablespoons of oat bran

- 3 tablespoons of low or zero fat Greek yogurt

Method

1. Whisk all the ingredients together to create a smooth batter, thinning with additional yogurt if required

2. Lightly oil a non-stick frying pan

3. Pour half of the mixture into the pan and cook until golden brown on each side

4. Repeat with the second part of the mixture

The basic galette, like the oat bran pancake can be made in bulk and frozen or refrigerated for up to a week.

Chapter 3

Lunchtime Meal Ideas and Recipes

Throughout the Dukan Diet it's important to continue to eat regularly and, as long as you stick to the allowed foods in each stage, you can eat as much as you like. Lunch, halfway through the day helps to boost your energy levels, keep your concentration levels high and will help to ward off the afternoon snack. In this chapter we look at suggested meal plans and recipes for lunch menus during the Attack Phase. Remember that as well as being suitable for PP days these recipes can be used at any time in the later stages of the diet either on PP days or with vegetables on PV days. Several of these meal plans and recipes will work well with oat bran galettes – see the previous chapter for a basic recipe.

Suggested Meal Plan

Day One

Baked Salmon Fillet with Dill

Cottage Cheese

Day Two

Spanish Style Seafood

Day Three

Cajun Mini-Burgers

Yogurt

Day Four

Thai Chicken or Turkey Patties

Day Five

Beef Kebabs

Day Six

Herby Omelet

Day Seven

Smoked Salmon on Basic Oat Bran Galette

Cottage Cheese

Lunchtime Recipes

Spanish Seafood Lunch

Ingredients (Serves 1)

- 1 packet of pre-cooked seafood mix

- Several drops of olive oil

- 1 Clove of garlic, crushed or chopped finely

- 1 teaspoon tomato puree

- 1/2 red chili, chopped

- Chives, chopped

- Salt and pepper

Method

1. Heat the oil in the pan and lightly brown the garlic

2. Add the seafood and once the water begins to evaporate add the chili, seasoning with salt and pepper to taste

3. Cook for 5 minutes before adding the tomato puree

4. Cook for a further 5 minutes, remove from the heat and stir in the chives.

Cajun Mini-Burgers

Ingredients (serves 2/3)

- 1.5 lb of lean chicken or turkey, minced
- 1 egg
- 2 tablespoons of oat bran
- 1 tablespoon of Cajun Spices
- 1 Green chili – finely chopped
- 2 cloves of garlic, crushed or chopped

Method

1. Mix the meat and other ingredients in a bowl, using a fork. You can also blend in a mixer for speed, if preferred

2. Shape the mixture into eight small balls and press to create burgers

3. Heat a pan with a little oil until hot

4. Cook the burgers until the meat is thoroughly cooked (around 15 – 20 minutes) turn regularly during cooking.

5. Serve with low fat or zero fat yogurt or cottage cheese

Herb Omelet

Ingredients

- 1 whole egg + 1 egg white

- 1 tablespoon of skimmed or low fat milk

- Chopped mixed herbs – your own favorites

- salt and pepper

Method

1. Gently mix the eggs and milk – to retain the color of yoke and white don't vigorously stir, just lightly break.

2. Add salt and pepper to taste

3. Heat a drop or two of oil in a frying pan

4. Add the mixture and then turn the heat to medium, cooking through and turning to brown both sides.

5. Serve on its own or with cottage cheese

Sharon Stone

Beef Kebabs

Ingredients (serves 2)

- 14oz Beef fillet
- 1tablespoon of cider vinegar
- ¼ of a cup of soy sauce (low-sodium)
- 2 tablespoons of Dijon mustard
- ¼ Cup of lemon juice
- Sprig of thyme and a bay leaf

Method

1. Cut the meat into good sized cubes

2. Mix the other ingredients in a large bowl – a baking dish is ideal

3. Add the meat to this marinade ensuring it's covered well and refrigerate for 4 hours (overnight for best results)

4. Place the meat on kebab skewers and grill turning regularly. Cook to your own preferences (medium, rare or well done)#

5. Serve alone or with low or zero fat Greek Yogurt as a dipping sauce

Thai Chicken or Turkey Patties with Greek Yogurt Dip

Ingredients (serves 2)

For the Patties

- 12oz of cooked chicken (this is a good recipe for using up leftovers)

- 1 clove of garlic, chopped finely

- 1 green chili, chopped roughly

- 1 piece of fresh ginger, chopped roughly

- ½ a red onion (or substitute with spring onions)

- 4 tablespoons of coriander

For the Dip

- 8oz of zero fat Greek Yogurt

- 2 tablespoons of chives, chopped

- 3 spring onions, chopped

- A dash of lemon, or lime, juice

- Salt and pepper

Method

Sharon Stone

1. For the dip simply use a blender to mix all the ingredients together. You can make this in advance, cover with cling-film and store in the refrigerator

2. For the patties, again, blend all the ingredients together until thoroughly mixed. Shape into patties using your hands – the mix should be enough to make six small patties

3. Lightly oil a non-stick pan and gently cook the chicken/turkey patties until brown. Ensure the meat is heated through completely, as it's already cooked this should take five minutes each side

4. Serve with your preprepared dip!

Chapter 4

Evening Meal Plans and Recipes

During the Attack Phase of the Dukan Diet you'll be restricted to protein rich foods, which may seem an expensive option – given that fresh meat and fish can often come at a higher cost. However, lunches and some breakfasts can be based on 'left-overs' from your main evening meal which helps to make the Attack Phase economical. In this chapter we look at a meal plan that allows for variety and also leaves some left over chicken for patties or burgers, or beef for skewers. Try to use fresh produce where possible and, if you can, buy organic meat. This is, in general, a much healthier approach to eating and as you progress through the stages of the diet you'll become used to cooking your own meals – which is good practice for the future. Remember all of these recipes can also be used on PV days in combination with allowed vegetables.

Dinner/Evening Meal Menu Plan

Day One

Rosemary Beef Burgers and Greek Yogurt Dip

Day Two

Teriyaki Tuna and Tzatziki

Day Three

Sea Bass in Herby Oat Bran Crust

Day Four

Cheesy Ham and Chicken Kiev

Day Five

Meatloaf

Day Six

Piri Piri Chicken

Day Seven

Rosemary Lemon Chicken

Dinner/Evening Meal Recipes

Rosemary Beef Burgers

Ingredients (serves 2)

For the Burgers

- 16oz lean beef mince

- 1 egg

- 3 tablespoons of oat bran

- 2 tablespoon of fresh rosemary, chopped

- 1 teaspoon of nutmeg

- black pepper

For the Dip

- 8oz of low, or zero, fat Greek Yogurt

- 1 teaspoon of smoked paprika

- 2 teaspoons of dried dill or handful of fresh

Method

1. For the dip simply mix the ingredients together thoroughly, cover with cling-film and place in the refrigerator

2. For the burgers mix all the ingredients together in a food processor and blitz until they are combined

3. Shape into small burgers with your hands – the mix should make 10 small burgers

4. Heat a non-stick pan until very hot and add the burgers, cook until meat is completely cooked through and the burgers are browned. Turn regularly during the process

5. Serve the burgers while hot along with the dip

Teriyaki Tuna with Tzatziki

Ingredients (serves 2)

- 2 Tuna Steaks

For the marinade

- 2 tablespoons of Teriyaki sauce
- 1 lime, juiced
- Black pepper

For the Tzatziki (Although this is the Attack Phase you can use cucumber in this recipe or if you prefer simply substitute with mint)

- 8oz of low, or zero, fat Greek Yogurt
- 1/3 of a cucumber de-seeded and chopped (or good handful of fresh mint, chopped)
- ½ clove of garlic, crushed
- ½ lemon – juiced
- 2 tablespoons of fresh dill
- salt and pepper

Method

1. Mix the Teriyaki sauce and lime juice together in a bowl and place the Tuna steaks in the bowl to

marinade – coat them carefully and allow to marinade for at least 30 minutes to 1 hour

2. While the Tuna is marinading blitz the cucumber (or mint), garlic, lemon juice and dill to a form a paste. Add the paste to a bowl with the Greek yogurt and combine all the ingredients together. Set aside in the refrigerator until ready to serve.

3. When the Tuna has had time to absorb the flavors, heat a pan with a little oil and add the steaks. Cooking times depend on your own taste – for rare 2 minutes each side should be plenty of time. Slightly longer for well done steaks is fine but Tuna dries out quickly so limit the time to no more than 4 minutes each side

4. Serve with the Tzatziki dip

Sea Bass in Herby Oat Bran Crust

Ingredients   (Serves   2)

- 4 Sea Bass Fillets

- 3 tablespoons of Oat Bran

- 2 tablespoons of water

- Fresh parsley – a good handful – chopped

- 2-3 sprigs of thyme

- Ground black pepper to tastes

- Olive oil

Method

1. If you have an oven-grill setting heat to 180C. If not use the grill only. While the grill is heating line a baking tray with grease proof paper, placing the Sea Bass fillets on this, skin side down

2. For the Oat Bran Crust mix the water, oat bran, herbs and seasoning in a bowl, mixing together with a fork. The mixture should quickly begin to look like coarse breadcrumbs

3. Spread the mixture on the fillets and spray with a touch of olive oil

4. Cook for 12-14 minutes in the middle of the oven and then move to the top of the oven to grill finally for a few minutes until golden brown.

Cheesy Ham and Chicken Kiev

Ingredients (serves 1 – double up the amounts for 2 servings)

- 1 – 2 tablespoons of low, or zero, fat cream cheese

- 1 skinned and boned chicken breast

- 1 slice of lean ham

- 1 teaspoon of chives, finely chopped (alternatively you can use garlic)

- Salt and pepper

Method

1. Carefully cut into the chicken breast to create a pocket

2. Mix the chives (or garlic) with the cream cheese and stuff into the pocket in the chicken (be careful not to overfill)

3. Season with salt and pepper and then wrap the chicken in the ham – covering the opening to the pocket.

4. Wrap in foil and cook in a preheated oven at 180C for 30 minutes

5. When cooked, unwrap the chicken and place under a grill to brown gently – you may need

cocktail sticks to keep the ham in place for this final part of the cooking.

Meatloaf

Ingredients (serves 6 and can be stored in the refrigerator, eaten cold or added to your lunch-box)

- 2lbs of lean minced beef

- 1 onion, chopped finely

- 2 eggs, beaten

- 4 tablespoons of low-fat fromage frais (yogurt can be substituted)

- 2 sliced hard boiled eggs

- Salt and pepper to season

Method

1. Preheat the oven 180C

2. Mix the beef, onion, the beaten eggs and fromage frais together carefully, seasoning with salt and pepper

3. Lightly oil a 2lb bread tin and dust with oat or wheat bran flour

4. Add *half* the mix into the tin and top with the sliced, boiled eggs

5. Add the remaining mix to the tin

6. Bake for 1 hour (you can turn the heat up for the last 5-10 minutes if you like a crusty brown top to the meatloaf)

Piri-Piri Chicken

Ingredients (serves 4)

- 4 skinned, boned chicken breast fillets or 8 skinned drumsticks

- The juice of ½ of a lemon and ½ a lime

- 2 Cloves of finely chopped garlic

- 2 teaspoons of crushed red chilis

- 1 teaspoon of paprika (hot or smoked to taste)

- 1 teaspoon of oregano

- ¼ cup of cider vinegar

- salt and pepper

Method

1. Mix the chilis, garlic, lemon, paprika, oregano and vinegar in a bowl to create the marinade

2. Add the chicken pieces ensuring they are thoroughly coated with the marinade

3. Cover the bowl with cling-film and leave to marinade overnight

4. After removing the chicken from the bowl season with salt and pepper

5. Turn the grill to a medium heat and grill till the chicken is thoroughly cooked and piping hot

6. Serve with plain yogurt and a drizzle of lime juice

Rosemary Lemon Chicken

Ingredients

- 1 Chicken (organic, free-range if possible)

- 4 Sprigs of Rosemary

- 4 Slices of Lemon

Method

1. Preheat your oven to 180C

2. Carefully using a sharp knife slit the skin of the chicken breast to create pockets and stuff 2 slices of lemon and 2 sprigs of rosemary into these pockets. Do the same on the underside of the chicken

3. Cover with foil and place in the oven to cook (check packaging for times). Once the chicken is cooked remove the skin and serve!

Chapter 5

Snack Attack Ideas and Additional Treats

For anybody on a diet the snack attack is a well known phenomenon. During the Attack Phase of the Dukan diet snacking can be a problem as there are no handy vegetables to fill that gap. Here are some suggestions for appropriate snack food during the Attack Phase, as well as two handy little recipes that you may find essential during the Attack Phase!

Dukan Diet Snack Ideas

- Beef, Game or Veal Jerky

- Hard boiled eggs

- Crab Sticks

- Smoked Salmon, rolled and filled with cream or cottage cheese

- Precooked seafood mixes

- Cooked prawns with yogurt or Greek style dip

- Roast chicken slices and Dukan mayonnaise

- Oat bran galettes (a real staple of the diet) filled with cream cheese, meat of your choice or smoked salmon

- Sugar free jelly

- Tinned tuna – in spring water or brine

Dukan Mayonnaise

Ingredients

- 3 tablespoons of low fat fromage frais or quark

- 1 tablespoon of Dijon mustard

- 1 egg yolk

- salt and pepper

Method

1. Beat the egg yolk gently in a bowl

2. Add the mustard, salt and pepper (you can also add paprika or very finely crushed garlic)

3. Add the fromage frais a small amount at a time, stirring continuously. If the mixture starts to curdle add a tiny splash of lemon juice and continue to mix carefully

4. When all the ingredients are combined you can use immediately but the mayonnaise can be kept in a sealed container in the refrigerator for several days

Dukan Chocolate Ice Cream

Note: Cocoa powder is not strictly speaking allowed at this stage in the diet but the small amount could be overlooked!

Ingredients

- 12oz of fat free fromage frais

- 3 separated eggs

- 6 teaspoons of granulated (but non-fructose) sweetener

- 2 teaspoons of reduced fat cocoa powder

- A dash of vanilla essence

Method

1. Use an electric whisk to mix the egg whites until they form stiff peaks and add the sweetener gradually during this process

2. Beat the yolks and add them to the whites stirring lightly

3. Add the cocoa powder and vanilla essence to the mixture and stir in lightly

4. In an ice cream maker churn until the mixture resembles soft ice cream (approximately 20 minutes)

5.   Enjoy! Although the mix can be stored for a week in a freezer, if you can resist that long!

Conclusion

Thank you again for buying this book!

I hope this book was able to inspire you during the first phase of the Dukan Diet.

The next step is to move on to the Cruise Phase of the diet. In this phase you will not lose weight as rapidly as during the Attack Phase, but gradually reducing your weight is healthier and allows both your body and your mind to adjust to your new eating habits.

Finally, if you enjoyed this book, please take the time to share your thoughts and post a review on Amazon. It'd be greatly appreciated!

Thank you and good luck!

Made in the USA
Middletown, DE
27 December 2022